# HERBAL REMEDIES FOR COMMON BLADDER ISSUES

Naturally Healing, Unlock The Power Of Holistic Solutions For Everyday Challenges

## DR. JEREMY ALLEY

## Disclaimer:

The information provided in this book, is intended for general informational purposes only and should not be considered as professional advice.

The author has made every effort to ensure the accuracy of the information presented. However, readers are advised to consult with a qualified healthcare professional before attempting any herbal remedies or making significant changes to their wellness routine. Individual health conditions vary, and what may be suitable for one person may not be appropriate for another.

It is important to note that the author is not in any endorsement deal, partnership, or affiliation with any organization, brand, or company mentioned in this book. Any references to specific products or services are based on the author's personal experience or general knowledge and do not imply an endorsement or promotion of those products or services.

# Contents

# Overview

Welcome to the investigation of herbal cures for urinary tract wellness. This trip explores the world of all-natural ways to support and preserve the health of your bladder. The bladder is an essential component of the urinary system and is vital for the removal of waste, therefore keeping it healthy is critical for general well-being.

## About The Book

Understanding how important bladder health is is crucial before diving into natural therapies. Urine is stored in the muscular organ known as the bladder until the body is ready to discharge it. When the bladder works at its best, waste is properly eliminated, which helps to avoid problems like UTIs and other related consequences.

Sufficient bladder health enhances a person's general quality of life by guaranteeing normal urination and lowering the chance of pain and infections. A person's food, lifestyle, and level of hydration can all have a big impact on their bladder's health. It is essential to comprehend these elements to choose the right herbal medicines and implement preventative measures.

The Function Of Herbal Treatments

For generations, people have used herbal treatments to treat a variety of health issues, including bladder health. A wide variety of plants found in nature have qualities that can support and improve bladder function. These treatments are frequently used because they can lessen inflammation, ease symptoms, and support a healthy urinary system.

Herbs related to bladder health include marshmallow root, uva-ursi, and maize silk.

Bearberry, or uva-ursi, is a plant that is known to have certain antibacterial qualities that may help treat and prevent urinary tract infections. Because of its well-known calming and anti-inflammatory properties, marshmallow root may help improve bladder comfort in general. The silky threads of corn ears are the source of corn silk, which has long been utilized to promote urinary tract health.

There are herbal combinations made especially for bladder health in addition to these individual herbs. These mixtures frequently contain different herbs with complementary qualities to address different elements of bladder function synergistically.

It is imperative to speak with a healthcare provider before introducing herbal treatments into a bladder health program, particularly if you are using medication or have pre-existing medical conditions. Herbal treatments are a great source of support, but they shouldn't be used in place of expert medical advice or care.

The subsequent sections will go deeper into the details of particular herbal treatments, including perspectives on their customary applications, possible advantages, and usage considerations. Come along on this herbal tour to learn about what nature has to offer in terms of preserving ideal bladder health.

The Structure And Operation Of The Bladder

Urine storage and elimination are critical functions of the bladder, an essential organ in the human urinary system. It is a muscle sac that is located in the pelvic cavity that contracts and expands as the urine is emptied. To understand the factors impacting bladder health, one must have a thorough understanding of the anatomy and function of the bladder.

An Overview Of The Bladder

A thorough understanding of the bladder entails investigating its composition, location, and main purposes. The kidneys, ureters, and urethra are all a part of the urinary tract, which also includes the bladder. Urine is primarily stored there until the body is ready to release it. The effectiveness of the bladder is essential for preserving general urinary health and averting several bladder-related problems.

The Bladder's Operation

The smooth operation of the bladder is dependent on the precise synchronization of sphincters, muscles, and nerves. The brain receives signals when the bladder fills with pee, alerting it to the need to empty. Urine flows out of the bladder when the sphincters, which function as valves, relax in response to the muscles in the bladder wall contracting. To treat any interruptions that can result in bladder health issues, it is essential to comprehend this complex mechanism.

Typical Bladder Health Problems

Numerous variables can affect bladder health, which can result in a variety of problems. Urinary incontinence, urinary tract infections (UTIs), bladder stones, and interstitial cystitis are common bladder health issues. These illnesses may result in pain, discomfort, and interruptions to regular activities. Investigating herbal treatments for bladder health becomes essential in treating and avoiding these problems, providing a holistic and all-natural way to keep the urinary system in good working order.

# CHAPTER ONE

## USE OF HERBS IN BLADDER HEALTH

A natural and comprehensive approach to maintaining bladder health is provided by herbal therapies. Keeping the bladder healthy is crucial for general well-being. These treatments can improve the general health of the urinary system and offer relief from frequent problems including urinary tract infections (UTIs).

### Herbal Remedies' Benefits

There are several advantages to using herbal treatments for bladder health. First of all, they frequently have antibacterial qualities that aid in the prevention or treatment of urinary tract infections. Furthermore, a lot of herbs have diuretic properties that help the body get rid of extra fluid and toxins. Herbal medicines are also well-known for their calming and anti-inflammatory qualities, which can help reduce bladder discomfort and irritation.

## Selecting The Correct Herbs

Making effective herbal treatments for bladder health requires a careful selection of the proper herbs. Every herb has special qualities that add to its overall health benefits. For bladder function support, it is important to take into account properties like antibacterial, diuretic, and anti-inflammatory actions while selecting herbs.

cranberry

Urinary tract infections can be prevented and treated with cranberries. It has substances that prevent bacteria from sticking to the walls of the urinary tract, lowering the chance of infection. Cranberries can be taken as a supplement or as juice to help maintain the health of the bladder.

Uva Ursi

Bearberry, or Uva Ursi, has long been used traditionally to treat urinary tract problems. It has substances like arbutin, which has antibacterial qualities and transforms into hydroquinone. Because of its possible advantages in supporting a healthy urinary system, uva ursi is frequently included in herbal blends or tinctures.

Dandelion Root

Prized for its diuretic qualities, dandelion root helps eliminate toxins and increases urine output. This herb may help support healthy bladder function overall and help avoid UTIs. You can drink dandelion root tea or take supplements.

Buchu

Native to South Africa, buchu is a herb valued for its anti-inflammatory and diuretic qualities. It has long been used to treat bladder irritation and urinary tract problems. There are several ways to include buchu in a bladder health program; it comes as teas and supplements, for example.

Cornflower

Another herbal cure for bladder health is cornsilk, which is the silky fiber found in corn cobs. It is prized for its calming qualities, which may lessen urinary tract inflammation. A comprehensive strategy for promoting bladder function may include the use of cornsilk, which is commonly made as a mild tea.

## Herbal Teas For Healthy Bladders

Herbal teas offer a tasty and practical means of supporting bladder health. Herbal blends that combine the aforementioned herbs with other health-promoting plants can provide a comprehensive strategy for preserving a healthy urinary system. Herbal teas are a great way to promote bladder health during uncomfortable periods or as a preventative step when sipped regularly.

Herbal therapies provide a comprehensive and natural substitute for conventional treatments when it comes to bladder health. Including these herbs in one's regimen, in the form of teas or supplements, can benefit the urinary system's general health, alleviate frequent ailments, and promote long-term well-being.

# CHAPTER TWO

## UPHOLDING AN HEALTHY STYLE

Adopting a healthy lifestyle is essential to maintaining good bladder health, which is critical for overall well-being. A comprehensive strategy takes into account several variables that affect bladder function, such as exercise, hydration, and food.

### The Value Of Hydration

Maintaining adequate hydration is essential for bladder health. Water aids in the removal of toxins from the body, avoiding the buildup of dangerous materials in the bladder. Additionally, it guarantees the effective operation of the urinary system, lowering the risk of infections and enhancing general urinary health.

### Nutritional Aspects

Bladder health is directly impacted by the food we eat. A nutritious and well-balanced diet can supply vital nutrients that support the urinary system. Foods high in fiber help promote regular bowel movements, which ward off constipation, which can strain the bladder.

## Foods That Support Healthy Bladders

Some foods are known to improve bladder health. Antioxidants found in berries, especially blueberries and cranberries, may help shield against UTIs. Incorporating vitamin C-rich foods, such as citrus fruits, can also maintain a healthy immune system, which in turn supports the bladder.

## Items To Steer Clear Of

Foods that can negatively affect bladder health exist in addition to those that support it. It is well known that caffeine, alcohol, and spicy meals irritate the bladder and can make symptoms worse for those who suffer from bladder disorders. Reducing the amount of these chemicals consumed can help keep the bladder healthy.

## Including Exercise To Maintain Bladder Health

Regular exercise is good for your health in general, including the operation of your bladder. Maintaining a healthy weight is facilitated by exercise, as it lowers the likelihood of disorders like obesity, which may exacerbate bladder problems. Kegel exercises are particularly useful for bladder health since they are specifically made to strengthen the muscles of the pelvic floor.

Maintaining the health of the bladder requires a multimodal strategy that includes food, exercise, and lifestyle decisions. People should take proactive measures to maintain normal bladder function and avoid future problems by drinking plenty of water, eating healthily, and exercising regularly.

# CHAPTER THREE

## HERBAL SOLUTIONS FOR REGULAR BLADDER ISSUES

Sustaining optimal bladder health is essential for overall health, and herbal medicines provide a holistic, natural solution for common bladder problems. Including herbal remedies in your routine can be helpful if you're trying to treat hyperactive bladder, avoid urinary tract infections (UTIs), manage interstitial cystitis, or reduce bladder inflammation.

### How To Avoid Utis (Urinary Tract Infections)

Urinary tract infections are a common issue that can be uncomfortable and interfere with day-to-day activities. Herbal treatments can be used as a component of a treatment strategy or as a preventative measure. Well-known for its ability to prevent UTIs by preventing bacteria from adhering to the walls of the urinary tract, cranberries are a beneficial herb. Other herbs that have been traditionally utilized for their diuretic and antibacterial qualities—which may help prevent UTIs—are dandelion root and uva-ursi.

A holistic strategy for preventing UTIs includes not only specific herbs but also regular hydration, basic cleanliness, and the adoption of lifestyle choices that boost immune function. Teas made from herbs, such as chamomile and green tea, can be incorporated into daily routines to support urinary health in general.

### Handling Cystitis Interstitial

The chronic bladder pain and discomfort associated with interstitial cystitis can have a major negative effect on a person's quality of life. Herbal treatments can reduce inflammation and soothe the inflamed bladder lining, which can provide comfort. The mucilage found in slippery elm and marshmallow root is well known for its ability to calm irritated tissues. Additionally, the anti-inflammatory qualities of herbs like ginger and turmeric may help to relieve the symptoms of interstitial cystitis.

A comprehensive strategy for treating interstitial cystitis includes nutritional adjustments, stress reduction, and pelvic floor exercises in addition to herbal therapies. Before using herbal medicines, it is best to speak with a healthcare provider, especially if you have a medical history or are currently taking other prescriptions.

## Natural Remedies For Hyperactive Bladder

Urinating frequently and urgently due to an overactive bladder might interfere with everyday activities. Herbal medicines can help treat the symptoms of an overactive bladder. Because saw palmetto can relax muscles, people with overactive bladders may benefit from using this herb, which has long been utilized to treat prostate health issues. In addition, studies have looked into the potential bladder-strengthening effects of horsetail and pumpkin seed extract.

Herbal remedies for overactive bladder are enhanced by addressing lifestyle issues, such as cutting back on caffeine and engaging in activities to train the bladder. As with any health issue, seeking advice from a medical specialist guarantees a customized and successful strategy.

## Natural Remedies For Inflammation Of The Bladder

Several things, such as irritants, infections, or autoimmune diseases, can cause bladder inflammation. Herbal treatments can provide a safe and effective way to lower inflammation and accelerate healing.

Native to South Africa, buchu is a plant with anti-inflammatory and diuretic qualities that may help relieve inflammation in the bladder. Another herb with diuretic properties, corn silk, may help reduce inflammation and help the body rid itself of impurities.

Including anti-inflammatory herbs like Boswellia and turmeric in one's diet helps promote a comprehensive approach to bladder inflammation management. The benefits of herbal medicines for bladder health are further enhanced by proper hydration, a balanced diet, and stress reduction.

Herbal treatments offer a wide range of all-natural solutions for bladder problems. Whether it's treating inflammation, controlling interstitial cystitis, curing hyperactive bladder, or preventing UTIs, the combination of herbal remedies and lifestyle changes can support an all-encompassing strategy for bladder health.

To guarantee the safety and effectiveness of herbal therapies, it is imperative to seek the advice of a healthcare practitioner.

# CHAPTER FOUR

## RECIPES AND FORMULAS USING HERBS

For general health, it is important to maintain optimal bladder health, and herbal therapies provide a safe, natural solution. For millennia, people have employed herbal recipes and formulae to promote bladder health and treat a variety of urinary disorders. These treatments use the therapeutic properties of plants to support healthy bladder function and reduce pain.

### Homemade Herbal Pelvic Health Tinctures

Making herbal tinctures for bladder health offers a customized, all-natural option. Herbal tinctures are concentrated liquid extracts that have therapeutic qualities. Use herbs like dandelion root, corn silk, and uva-ursi, which are known to have positive benefits on the urinary system, to produce a homemade tincture for bladder health. Mix these herbs to the appropriate strength and steep in a base of glycerin or high-proof alcohol. By extracting the active ingredients, a strong tincture that can be taken frequently to support bladder function is produced.

## Tears-Relieving Herbal Concoctions

Herbal infusions are a potent additional means of supporting bladder health. Maintaining a healthy urinary system can be achieved by incorporating calming herbs into your everyday routine. Herbs with bladder-calming effects such as marshmallow root, parsley, and chamomile have long been employed.

Steep these plants in hot water for a long time to extract their medicinal properties to make an herbal infusion.

Regular consumption of this herbal infusion can improve overall urinary wellness and bladder comfort.

## Herbal Concoctions For Elimination

Maintaining bladder health requires detoxification, which is why herbal blends created especially for this reason can be helpful.

Herbs with diuretic and detoxifying qualities include cleavers, dandelion leaf, and nettle. By combining these plants, you can take advantage of their synergistic properties by making a herbal blend.

This blend offers a mild yet efficient means of assisting the bladder's natural detoxification processes. It can be added to tinctures or infused into teas.

To sum up, herbal therapies provide a comprehensive and all-natural method of preserving bladder health.

Whether you use these herbal remedies in your daily routine for cleansing blends, calming infusions, or homemade tinctures, they can help maintain a stronger and healthier urinary system. Before making big changes to your health regimen, as with any regimen, it's best to speak with a healthcare provider, particularly if you take medication or have pre-existing medical conditions.

# CHAPTER FIVE

## INCLUDING HERBS IN EVERYDAY LIFE

A natural and comprehensive approach to supporting bladder health is provided by herbal treatments, which are essential for maintaining a healthy bladder for general well-being.

Since ancient times, traditional medical systems all around the world have employed herbs, demonstrating how well they can support a range of wellness-related issues.

Herbs are a very beneficial addition to your everyday routine when it comes to bladder health.

### Including Herbal Remedies In Your Daily Practice

Herbal treatments for bladder health can be included easily in everyday activities. Popular herbs including marshmallow root, horsetail, and uva ursi are well-known for their beneficial benefits on the bladder.

For example, uva ursi has antibacterial qualities that might help shield against urinary tract infections. In contrast, marshmallow root has a reputation for being calming and anti-inflammatory, which may help ease bladder irritation. Due to its high silica content, horsetail supports bladder function overall and aids in tissue healing.

Making herbal tinctures, infusing them into teas, or incorporating them into meals are easy ways to incorporate these herbs into your daily routine. Herbal teas can offer a calming and hydrating experience that encourages the best possible bladder function.

Incorporating these herbs into your diet through cooking or infusions also guarantees a steady intake, which supports long-term bladder health.

## Advice On Responsible And Sustainable Herb Use

To fully reap the benefits of herbal medicines for bladder health, it is imperative to use herbs sustainably and responsibly.

Think about growing your herbs at home to maintain a fresh and easily accessible supply while also building a relationship with the natural world. Choose reliable suppliers that value sustainability and moral harvesting methods when buying herbs.

It's important to know how much and how long to take herbal treatments. Seeking advice from a qualified herbalist or medical practitioner can offer tailored recommendations based on specific needs and health problems.

Consuming herbs responsibly involves knowing where they come from, how they are grown, and how their production affects the environment.

Although herbs can provide beneficial support for bladder health, one must be aware of possible side effects and precautions.

Certain herbs may have negative effects on specific medical problems or interact negatively with pharmaceuticals. For example, people with kidney problems should be careful while using herbs such as uva ursi, as they can make pre-existing diseases worse.

Before introducing herbal treatments into their routine, people who are pregnant or nursing should also speak with healthcare specialists, since certain herbs may not be appropriate during these times. To be sure that using herbal medicines complements your entire health plan, always reveal any current prescriptions or health issues.

Using the advantages of herbal medicines for bladder health requires incorporating herbs into everyday life, adhering to sustainable practices, and being cautious. Responsible use of these natural remedies can help people maintain their general health and bladder function.

# CHAPTER SIX

## SUCCESS STORIES

The testimonials from people who have had success with herbal medicines for bladder health are among the most persuasive features of these treatments. Those looking for natural and alternative ways to preserve and enhance bladder function will find inspiration in these stories. Success tales provide insight into the observable advantages of integrating herbal treatments into one's everyday regimen.

### Individual Testimonies

Understanding the effects of herbal treatments on bladder health depends critically on individual experiences with them. Testimonials from individuals offer firsthand experiences of people who have used herbal remedies in their daily routines. These tales provide hope and inspiration to people considering natural remedies by illuminating the various ways in which herbs might improve bladder function.

## Case Studies

This section delves deeper into the scientific and useful aspects of herbal medicines. It does this by examining case studies that look at the effectiveness of particular herbs in supporting bladder health. Readers get a more thorough grasp of how herbal remedies might treat different bladder-related illnesses by looking at real-world instances. Case studies provide empirically supported insights that broaden our understanding of natural bladder health strategies.

For anyone looking for information on herbal remedies for bladder health, this handbook is a great resource. This page's information, which includes case studies, success stories, and individual testimonies, attempts to inform and encourage readers as they embark on a journey to naturally maintain a healthy and functional bladder.

## Herbal Medicine's Power

Herbal therapy benefits from the complex biochemistry found in plants. Many herbs are effective partners in the fight against fungal infections and athlete's foot because of their antibacterial, anti-inflammatory, and antifungal qualities.

These substances produced from plants can enhance general foot health, aid in healing, and reduce discomfort. Knowing the distinct qualities of each plant enables people to customize their strategy to meet their requirements.

## Safety Points To Remember

Herbal treatments provide a safe and natural route to healthy feet, but caution must be exercised when using them. Potential allergies, drug combinations, and personal sensitivities are all safety concerns. Before starting a herbal regimen, speaking with a healthcare provider or herbalist can help to confirm that the treatments selected are appropriate for the individual's unique health profile.

For people who take medicine or have pre-existing medical conditions, this precaution is especially crucial.

## The Best Herbs To Use For Foot Health

An essential component of herbal foot care is choosing the appropriate herbs. Tea tree oil is a well-liked option because of its strong antifungal qualities. Applying it sparingly can help reduce symptoms and stop the growth of fungi.

Herbs with antibacterial and calming properties, such as calendula, lavender, and garlic, also add to the overall efficacy of herbal foot cures. A comprehensive and individualized approach to foot health can be created by being aware of the special advantages that each plant offers.

## CONCLUSION

To sum up, herbal treatments offer a strong, all-natural treatment for fungal infections and athlete's foot. Their all-encompassing approach, which includes relaxing, anti-inflammatory, and antibacterial qualities, can relieve pain and support general foot health. But exercise extreme caution, and speaking with a medical expert guarantees a customized and secure herbal regimen.

### Recap Of Herbal Remedies

A summary of herbal remedies demonstrates the wide variety of herbs that can be used to promote foot health. Herbs have different medicinal powers; some are strong antifungals like tea tree oil, while others have calming qualities like calendula and lavender. People can fully utilize herbal medicine for the best possible foot health by carefully combining these remedies.

## Gaining Self-Power Through Herbal Knowledge

Gaining herbal knowledge to empower oneself is a lifetime journey. A person can make educated decisions about their health by being aware of the characteristics, uses, and possible interactions of herbs.

Whether tackling particular foot issues or adopting a more comprehensive herbal way of life, lifelong learning guarantees that people may effectively and confidently traverse the enormous field of herbal medicine.